KETO COOKBOOK 2021

Easy Keto Recipes for Busy People to Keep A ketogenic Diet Lifestyle

Emily Cooper

Sommario

Breakfast Recipes

The Mocha Shake

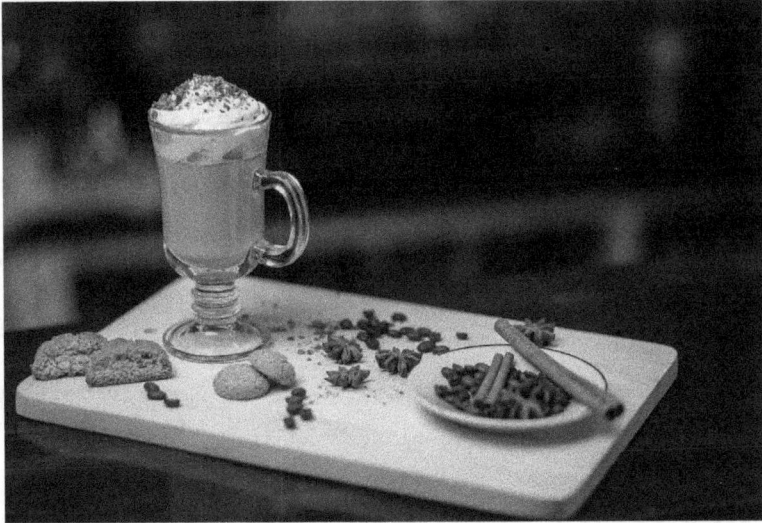

Serving: 1
Prep Time: 10 minutes
Ingredients:
- 1 cup whole milk
- 2 tablespoons cocoa powder
- 2 pack stevia
- 1 cup brewed coffee, chilled
- 1 tablespoon coconut oil

Directions:
1. Add listed ingredients to blender
2. Blend until you have a smooth and creamy texture
3. Serve chilled with some biscuits and muffins if you prefer, add Keto-Friendly whipped cream on top if desired
4. Enjoy!

Nutritional Contents:

- Calories: 293
- Fat: 23g
- Carbohydrates: 19g
- Protein: 10g

Early Morning Cheesy Egg Muffin

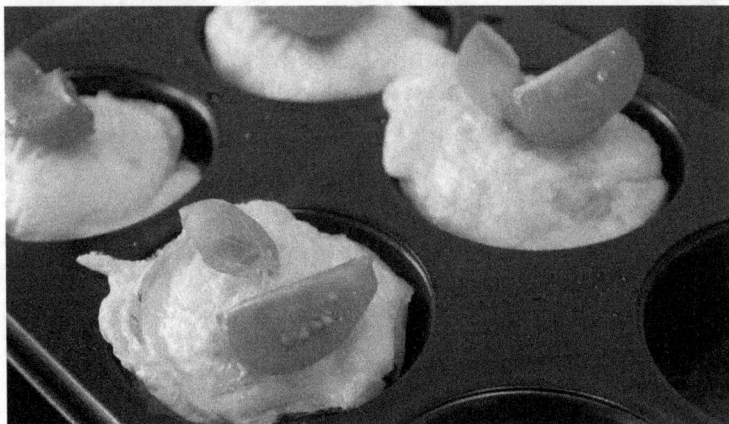

Serving: 6
Prep Time: 10 minutes
Cook Time: 20 minutes

Ingredients

- 4 large whole eggs
- 2 tablespoons Greek yogurt
- Salt and pepper taste
- 3 tablespoons coconut flour
- ¼ teaspoon baking powder
- ½ cup cheddar cheese, shredded

How To

1. Pre-heat your oven to 375-degree F

2. Add yogurt, eggs to a medium sized bowl

3. Season with salt and pepper, whisk well

4. Add baking powder, coconut flour and mix until you have a smooth batter

5. Add cheese and fold

6. Pour mix evenly in 6 silicone muffin cups and bake in your oven until golden

7. Enjoy!

Nutrition (Per Serving)

- Calories: 101
- Fat: 7g
- Carbohydrates: 3g
- Protein: 7g

An Omelet Of Swiss Chard

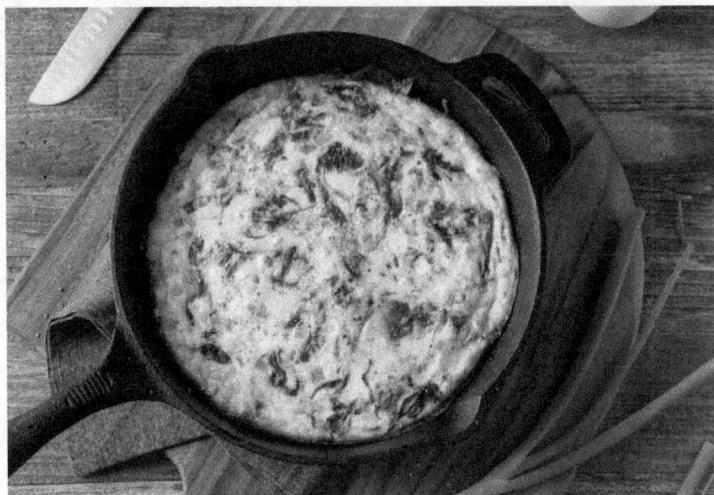

Serving: 4
Prep Time: 5 minutes
Cook Time: 5 minutes

Ingredients

- 4 eggs, lightly beaten
- 4 cups Swiss chard, sliced
- 2 tablespoons butter
- ½ teaspoon garlic salt
- Fresh pepper

How To

1. Take a non-stick frying pan and place it over medium-low heat
2. Once the butter melts, add Swiss chard and stir cook for 2 minutes
3. Pour egg into pan and gently stir them into Swiss chard
4. Season with garlic salt and pepper
5. Cook for 2 minutes
6. Serve and enjoy!

Nutrition (Per Serving)

- Calories: 260
- Fat: 21g
- Carbohydrates: 4g
- Protein: 14g

Chocolate Fat Bombs

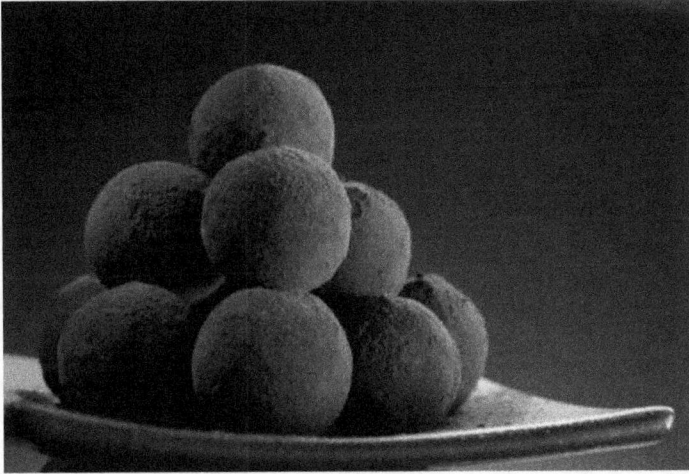

Serving: 12 balls
Prep Time: 10 minutes + chill time
Cook Time: 5 minutes

Ingredients

- ¾ cup coconut oil
- 1 cup almond butter
- 1/3 cup cocoa powder
- ¼ cup almond, ground
- ½ teaspoon salt
- Stevia if needed

How To

1. Add listed ingredients to pot and place over low heat, stir until everything melts

2. Once the mixture is combined and forms a thick batter, let it cool

3. Roll mixture into balls and place on a paper lined baking tray

4. Place tray into fridge and let them cool for 1 hour

5. Serve and enjoy!

Nutrition (Per Serving)

- Calories: 555
- Fat: 55g
- Carbohydrates: 11g
- Protein: 11g

Coconut And Hazelnut Chilled Glass

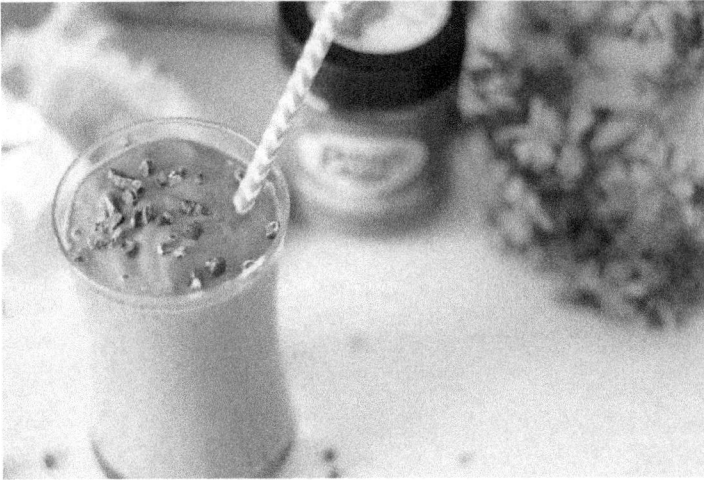

Serving: 1
Prep Time: 10 minutes

Ingredients:

- ½ cup coconut milk
- ¼ cup hazelnuts, chopped
- 1 and ½ cups water
- 1 pack stevia

Directions:

1. Add listed ingredients to blender

2. Blend until you have a smooth and creamy texture

3. Serve chilled and enjoy!

Nutritional Contents:

- Calories: 457
- Fat: 46g
- Carbohydrates: 12g
- Protein: 7g

Appetizer and Snacks Recipes

Golden Eggplant Fries

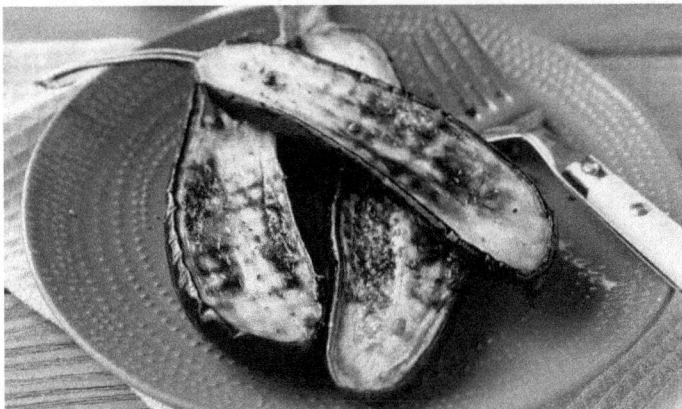

Serving: 8
Prep Time: 10 minutes
Cook Time: 15 minutes

Ingredients
- 2 eggs
- 2 cups almond flour
- 2 tablespoons coconut oil, spray
- 2 eggplant, peeled and cut thinly
- Salt and pepper

How To

1. Preheat your oven to 400 degree Fahrenheit
2. Take a bowl and mix with salt and black pepper in it
3. Take another bowl and beat eggs until frothy
4. Dip the eggplant pieces into eggs
5. Then coat them with flour mixture
6. Add another layer of flour and egg
7. Then, take a baking sheet and grease with coconut oil on top
8. Bake for about 15 minutes
9. Serve and enjoy!

Nutrition (Per Serving)

- Calories: 212
- Fat: 15.8g
- Carbohydrates: 12.1g
- Protein: 8.6g

Cheesy Mozzarella Sticks

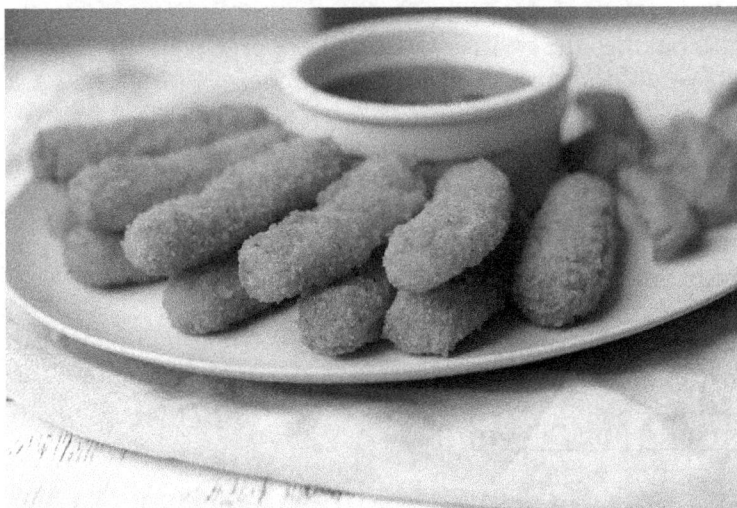

Serving: 8 bread sticks
Prep Time: 10 minutes
Cook Time: 20 minutes

Ingredients
- 2 cups shredded mozzarella cheese
- 2 tablespoons coconut flour
- 2 whole eggs
- 1 pinch of salt

Toppings
- ½ cup shredded parmesan cheese
- 1 tablespoons Italian seasoning
- ½ teaspoon garlic powder

How To

1. Pre-heat your oven to 350 degree F
2. Line a baking sheet with parchment paper
3. Take your food processor and add cheese, flour, eggs, salt and process
4. Scoop the mix onto your lined baking sheet and flatten to 1 inch thickness, forming a square
5. Bake for 15 minutes
6. Remove from oven and sprinkle parmesan cheese, Italian seasoning and garlic powder
7. Bake for 5 minutes
8. Remove from oven and let it cool
9. Serve and enjoy!

Nutrition (Per Serving)

- Calories: 225
- Fat: 19g
- Carbohydrates: 3g
- Protein: 12g

Salt And Rosemary Cracker

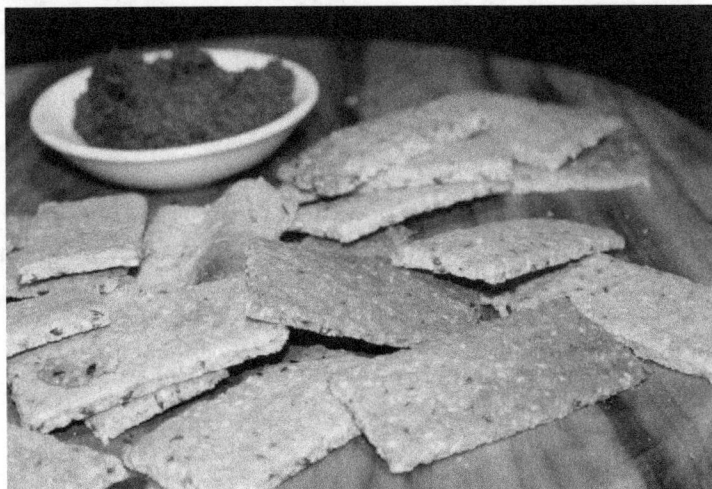

Serving: 36 Crackers
Prep Time: 10 minutes
Cook Time: 10-15 minutes

Ingredients

- 1 and ½ cups almond flour
- ½ teaspoon Celtic salt
- 1 egg, at room temp
- 2 tablespoons coconut oil
- ¼ teaspoon pepper
- 1 tablespoon rosemary, chopped

How To

1. Pre-heat oven to 350 degree F
2. Take a baking tray and line it with parchment paper
3. Take a bowl and add almond flour, salt and keep it on the side
4. Take another bowl and add coconut oil, pepper, rosemary
5. Add almond mix to the bowl
6. Mix well until you have an even dough
7. Transfer dough to a piece of parchment paper, cover with another parchment paper piece and roll it out into a thin layer
8. Cut into crackers, arrange them on prepped baking sheet
9. Bake for 10-15 minutes
10. Let them cool
11. Serve and enjoy!

Nutrition (Per Serving)

- Calories: 66
- Fat: 6g
- Carbohydrates: 1.4g
- Protein: 3g

Premium Goat Cheese Salad

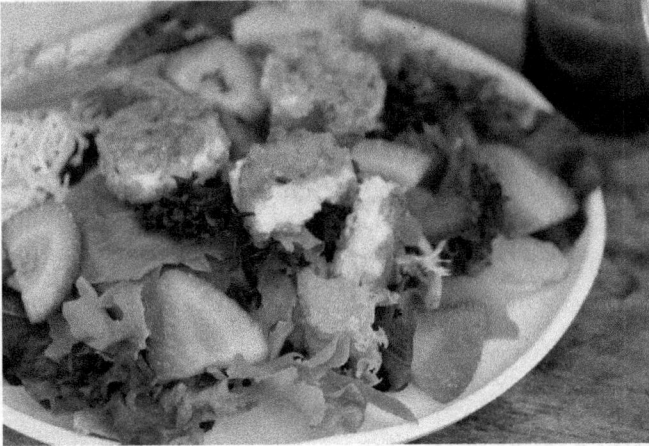

Serving: 2
Prep Time: 4 minutes
Cook Time: 10 minutes

Ingredients

- 1 and ½ cups Hard Goat cheese, grated
- 4 cups spinach, fresh
- 4 strawberries, garnish
- ½ cup flaked almonds, toasted
- 4 tablespoons Raspberry vinaigrette, check for Keto-Friendliness

How To

1. Pre-heat your oven to 400 degree F

2. Line a baking sheet using parchment paper, cut the parchment paper in half

3. Grate goat cheese onto each half

4. Form two circles using the grated cheese

5. Bake for 10 minutes

6. Transfer to a bowl and let it cool in the bowl shape

7. Peel the cheese off

8. Add remaining ingredients into the cheese and toss well

9. Serve immediately and enjoy!

Nutrition (Per Serving)

- Calories: 645
- Fat: 53g
- Carbohydrates: 6g
- Protein: 33g

Grilled Avocado And Melted Cheese

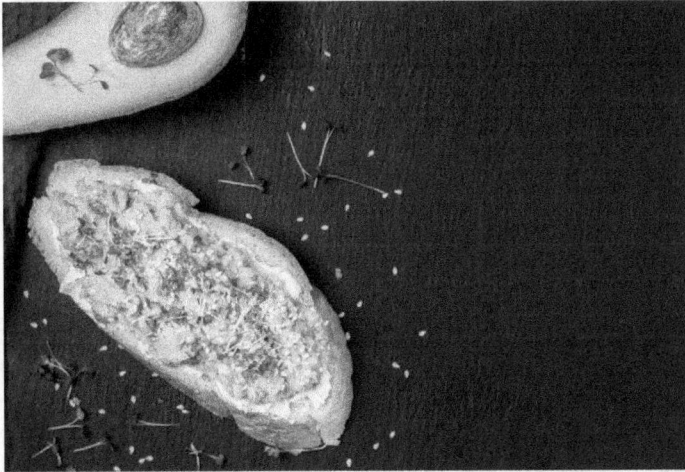

Serving: 6
Prep Time: 5 minutes
Cook Time: 4 minutes

Ingredients

- 1 whole avocado
- 1 tablespoon chipotle sauce
- 1 tablespoon lime juice
- ¼ cup parmesan cheese
- Salt and pepper to taste

How To

1. Prepare avocado by slicing half lengthwise, and discard seed

2. Gently prick skin of avocado with fork

3. Set your avocado halves, skin down on small baking sheet, lined with aluminum foil

4. Top with sauce and drizzle lime juice

5. Season with salt and pepper

6. Sprinkle half parmesan cheese in each cavity, set your broiler to high for 2 minutes

7. Add rest of the cheese and return to your broiler until cheese melts and avocado slightly browns

8. Serve hot and enjoy!

Nutrition (Per Serving)

- Calories: 459
- Fat: 41g
- Carbohydrates: 15g
- Protein: 7g

Beef Recipes

Pure Broccoli Rib Eye

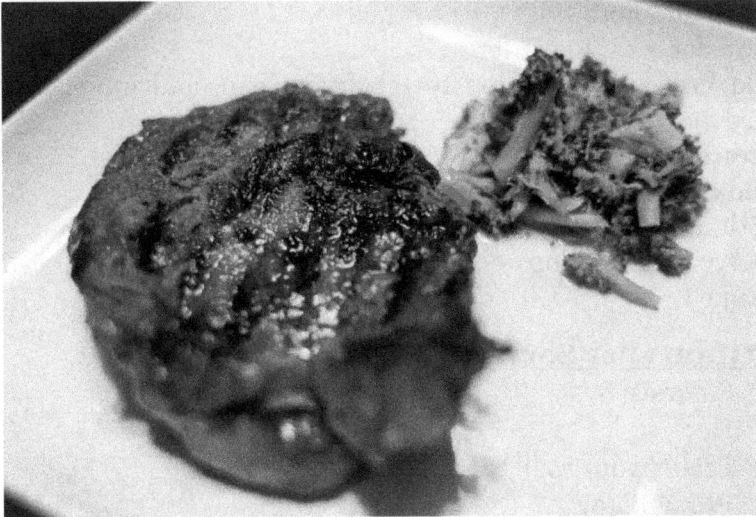

Serving: 4
Prep Time: 5 minutes
Cook Time: 15 minutes

Ingredients

- 4 ounces butter
- ¾ pound Ribeye steak, sliced
- 9 ounces broccoli, chopped
- 1 yellow onion, sliced
- 1 tablespoon coconut aminos
- 1 tablespoon pumpkin seeds
- Salt and pepper to taste

How To

1. Slice steak and the onions

2. Chop broccoli, including the stem parts

3. Take a frying pan and place it over medium heat, add butter and let it melt

4. Add meat and season accordingly with salt and pepper

5. Cook until both sides are browned

6. Transfer meat to platter

7. Add broccoli and onion to the frying pan, add more butter if needed

8. Brown

9. Add coconut aminos and return the meat

10. Stir and season again

11. Serve with a dollop of butter with a sprinkle of pumpkin seeds

12. Enjoy!

Nutrition (Per Serving)

- Calories: 875
- Fat: 75g
- Carbohydrates: 8g
- Protein: 40g

Cilantro And Lime Skirt Steak

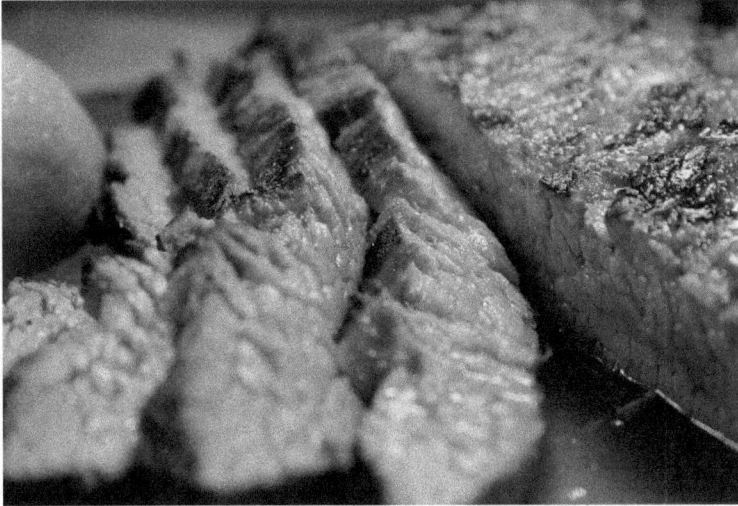

Serving: 3
Prep Time: 45 minutes
Cook Time: 10 minutes
<u>Ingredients</u>
For the Cilantro Lime Steak Marinade
- 1 pound of Skirt Steak
- ¼ cup of coconut aminos
- ¼ cup of Olive Oil
- 1 medium sized lime, juiced
- 1 teaspoon of garlic, minced
- 1 small sized Handful Cilantro
- ¼ teaspoon of Red Pepper Flakes

For the Cilantro Paste
- 1 teaspoon of garlic, minced
- ½ a teaspoon of Salt
- 1 cup of lightly fresh cilantro
- ¼ cup of olive oil
- ½ a medium sized lemon, juiced

- 1 medium sized deseeded Jalapeno
- ½ a teaspoon of Cumin
- ½ a teaspoon of Coriander

How To

1. Remove the outer silver skin off the skirt steak
2. Take a plastic bag and add the Cilantro Lime Steak marinade ingredients to the bag, add the steak and mix to coat it up
3. Allow it to marinate for 45 minutes in your fridge
4. Make the sauce by adding the paste ingredients to a food processor and pulse until blended to a paste
5. Take an iron skillet and place it over medium-high heat
6. Remove the steak from the bag transfer steak to the pan and sear both sides (each side for 2-3 minutes)
7. Serve with the cilantro sauce on top
8. Enjoy!

Nutrition(Per Serving)

- Calories: 432
- Fat: 32g
- Carbohydrates: 4g
- Protein: 38g

Mushroom And Olive "Mediterranean" Steak

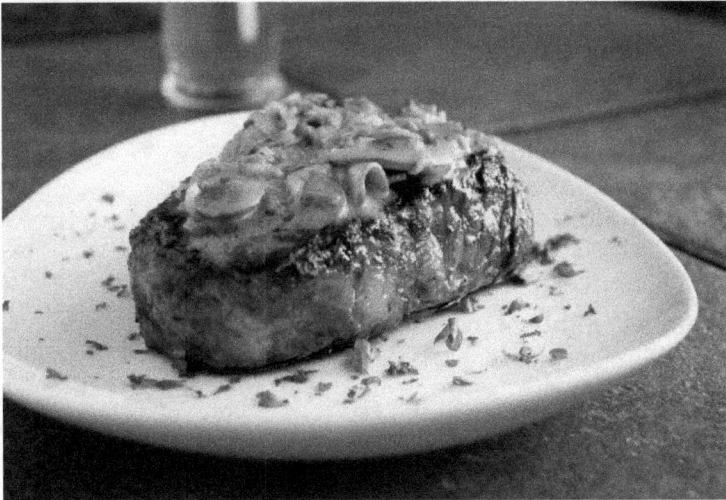

Serving: 4
Prep Time: 10 minutes
Cook Time: 14 minutes

Ingredients

- 1 pound boneless beef sirloin steak, ¾ inch thick, cut into 4 pieces
- 1 large red onion, chopped
- 1 cup mushrooms
- 4 garlic cloves, thinly sliced
- 4 tablespoons olive oil
- ½ cup green olives, coarsely chopped
- 1 cup parsley leaves, finely cut

How To

1. Take a large sized skillet and place it over medium high heat
2. Add oil and let it heat p
3. Add beef and cook until both sides are browned, remove beef and drain fat
4. Add rest of the oil to skillet and heat I up
5. Add onions, garlic and cook for 2-3 minutes
6. Stir well
7. Add mushrooms olives and cook until mushrooms are thoroughly done
8. Return beef to skillet and lower heat to medium
9. Cook for 3-4 minutes (covered_
10. Stir in parsley
11. Serve and enjoy!

Nutrition (Per Serving)

- Calories: 386
- Fat: 30g
- Carbohydrates: 11g
- Protein: 21g

Satisfying Low-Carb Beef Liver Salad

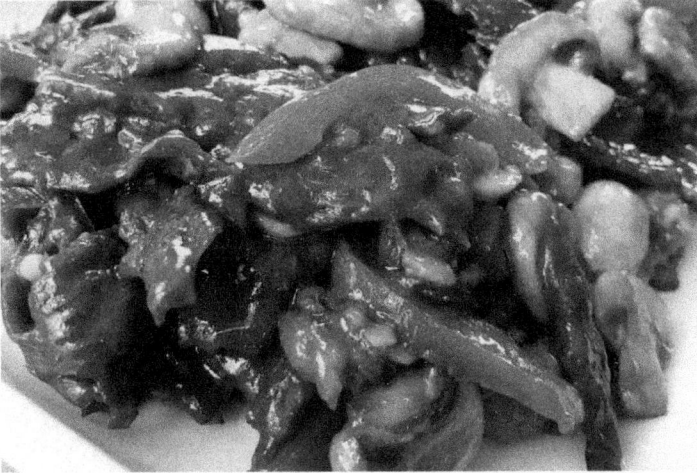

Serving: 3
Prep Time: 10 minutes
Cook Time: Nil

Ingredients
- 3-4 ounces beef liver, cooked
- 1 egg, hard boiled
- 1 ounce dried mushroom
- 1 whole onion, minced
- 2 ounces mayonnaise
- 2 ounces olive oil
- Salt and pepper to taste
- Dill for serving
- ½ a red bell pepper, sliced

How To
1. Cut mushroom and livers into strips and transfer to a bowl
2. Peel the egg and slice it, transfer to bowl
3. Add remaining ingredients and toss well
4. Sprinkle with dill and serve!

Nutrition (Per Serving)
- Calories: 300
- Fat: 26g
- Carbohydrates: 5g
- Protein: 10g

Perfect Aromatic Beef Roast

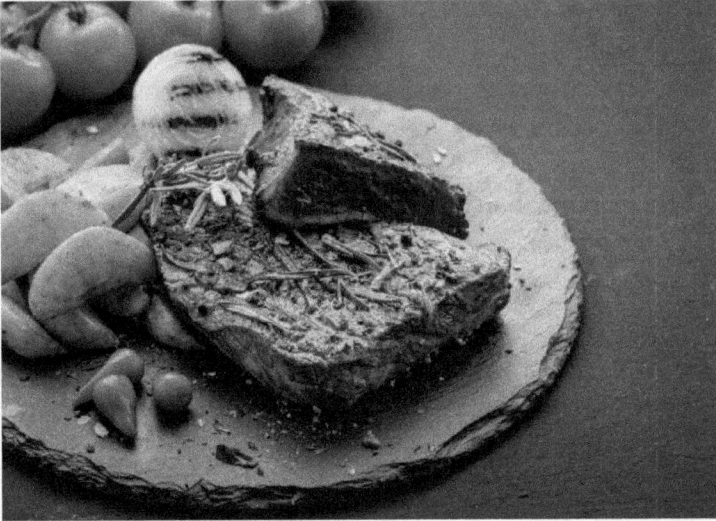

Serving: 4
Prep Time: 10 minutes
Cook Time: 50 minutes

Ingredients

- 1 lb of beef sirloin or similar lean cut for roast
- 2 tbsp of mustard
- 2 tbsp of olive oil
- 2 tbsp of garlic salt
- 1 spring of fresh rosemary

How To

1. Combine the mustard, olive oil, and garlic salt in a small bowl.

2. Take the roast beef, remove excess fat and make small incisions lengthwise so you can let the mixture penetrate more easily.

3. Brush the mustard mixture over the beef, making sure it all nicely coated.

4. Place on a baking dish and arrange the rosemary leaves on the sides for extra aroma.

5. Cook in a preheated oven at 380F/180 C for 50 minutes (for a medium cook inside).

6. Serve with mashed sweet potatoes and/or salad

Nutrition (Per Serving)

- Calories: 646
- Fat: 27g
- Carbohydrates: 0.1g
- Protein: 96g

Pork And Other Read Meat

Gentle Cheesy Pork Chops

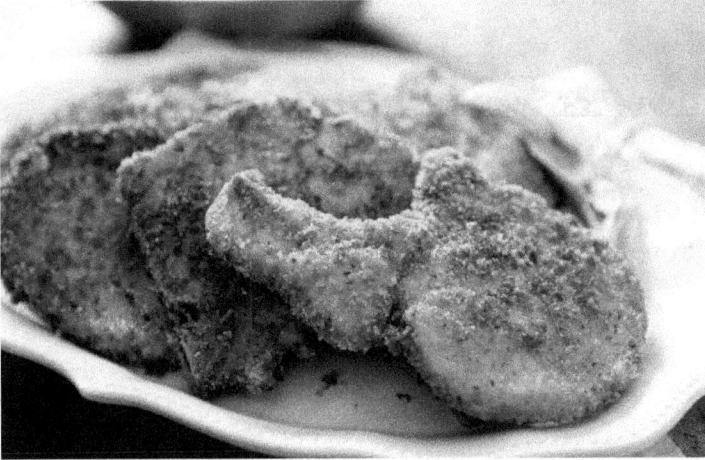

Serving: 4
Prep Time: 10 minutes
Cook Time: 20 minutes

Ingredients

- 3 ounces parmesan cheese
- ½ cup almond flour
- 7 center cut, pork chops
- 1 whole egg
- Bacon grease for frying
- Salt and pepper to taste

How To
1. Pre-heat your oven to 400-degree F
2. Take a bowl and mix in cheese, flour and seasoning
3. Take another bowl and mix in egg
4. Dip pork chops in eggs, followed by a dip in the flour /cheese mix
5. Fry in oil for 1-2 minutes each side (on medium heat)
6. Transfer to a baking dish and bake in oven until golden brown
7. Enjoy!

Nutrition (Per Serving)
- Calories: 350
- Fat: 35g
- Carbohydrates: 4g
- Protein: 31g

Original Caramelized Pork Chops

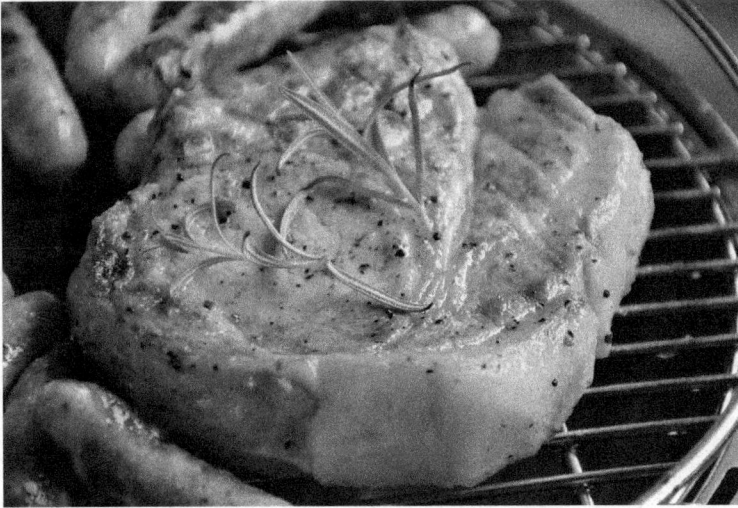

Serving: 4
Prep Time: 5 minutes
Cook Time: 30 minutes

Ingredients

- 4 pounds chuck roast
- 4 ounces green chili, chopped
- 2 tablespoons chili powder
- ½ teaspoon dried oregano
- ½ teaspoon ground cumin
- 2 garlic cloves, minced
- Salt as needed

How To

1. Rub up your chop with 1 teaspoon of pepper and 2 teaspoon of seasoning salt

2. Take a skillet and heat some oil over medium heat

3. Brown your pork chops on each sides

4. Add water and onions to the pan

5. Cover it up and lower down the heat, simmer it for about 20 minutes

6. Turn your chops over and add the rest of the pepper and salt

7. Cover it up and cook until the water evaporates and the onions turn to a medium brown texture

8. Remove the chops from your pan and serve with some onions on top!

Nutrition (Per Serving)

- Calories: 271
- Fat: 19g
- Carbohydrates: 4g
- Protein: 27g

Simple Pork Stuffed Bell Peppers

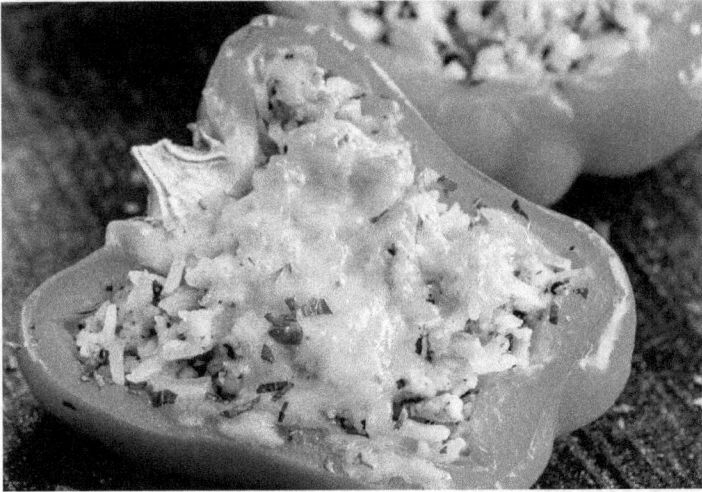

Serving: 4
Prep Time: 10 minutes
Cook Time: 26 minutes

Ingredients

- 1 teaspoon Cajun spice
- 1 pound pork, ground
- 1 tablespoons tomato paste
- 6 garlic cloves, minced
- 1 yellow onion, chopped
- 4 big bell peppers, tops cut off and deseeded
- Pinch of salt
- Black pepper as needed
- 1 cup cheddar cheese

How To

1. Take a pan and place it over medium-high heat
2. Add oil and let the oil heat up
3. Add garlic, onion and cook for 4 minutes
4. Add meat and gently stir cook for 10 minutes
5. Season with salt and pepper according to your desire
6. Add Cajun seasoning and tomato paste
7. Stir cook for 3 minutes more
8. Stuff bell peppers with the mix and transfer to a pre-heated grill, top with cheese
9. Grill for 3 minutes (each side)
10. Divide between plates and serve
11. Enjoy!

Nutrition (Per Serving)

- Calories: 140
- Fat: 3g
- Carbohydrates: 3g
- Protein: 10g

Parmesan Pork Steak

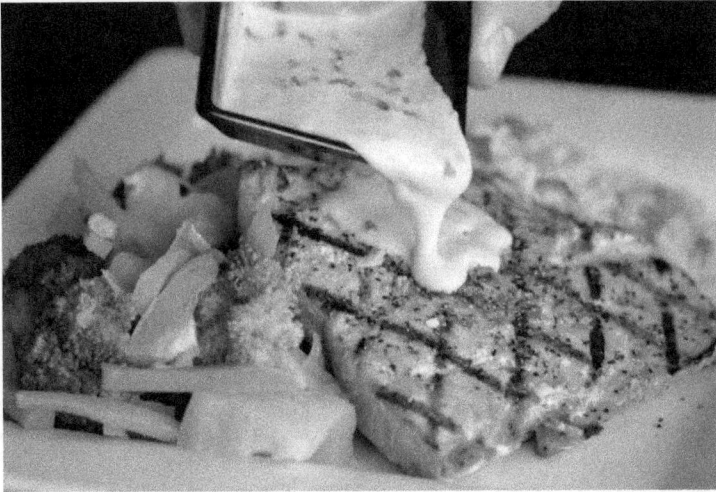

Serving: 4
Prep Time: 10 minutes
Cook Time: 15 minutes

Ingredients

- ½ pound pork steak
- Salt and pepper to taste
- 1 ounce parmesan, grated/melted
- 1 tablespoon lemon juice
- 2 tablespoons olive oil

How To

1. Beat the pork steak with kitchen mallet to flatten it a bit
2. Season with salt and pepper
3. Let it rest for a few minutes
4. Take a frying pan and grease it with oil, place it over high heat
5. Once the oil is hot, add steak and cook for 7-8 minutes per side
6. Transfer cooked steak on a plate and drizzle lemon juice
7. Cover with grated parmesan/melted parmesan
8. Serve and enjoy!

Nutrition (Per Serving)

- Calories: 315
- Fat: 27g
- Carbohydrates: 1g
- Protein: 16g

Curious Slow Cooked Cranberry And Pork Roast

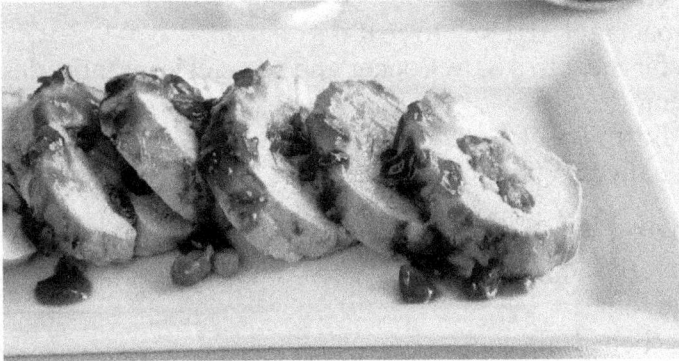

Serving: 4
Prep Time: 10 minutes
Cook Time: 8 hours

Ingredients

- 1 tablespoon coconut flour
- Salt and pepper to taste
- 1 and ½ pound pork loin
- Pinch of dry mustard
- ½ teaspoon ginger
- 2 tablespoons stevia
- ½ cup cranberries
- 2 garlic cloves, peeled and minced
- ½ lemon, sliced
- ¼ cup water

How To
1. Take a owl and add ginger, mustard, pepper and flour
2. Stir well
3. Add roast and toss well to coat it
4. Transfer meat to a Slow Cooker and add stevia, cranberries, garlic, water, lemon slices
5. Place lid and cook on LOW for 8 hours
6. Drizzle the pan juice on top and serve!

Nutrition (Per Serving)
- Calories: 430
- Fat: 23g
- Carbohydrates: 3g
- Protein: 45g

Poultry Recipes

Chicken Parmesan Fingers

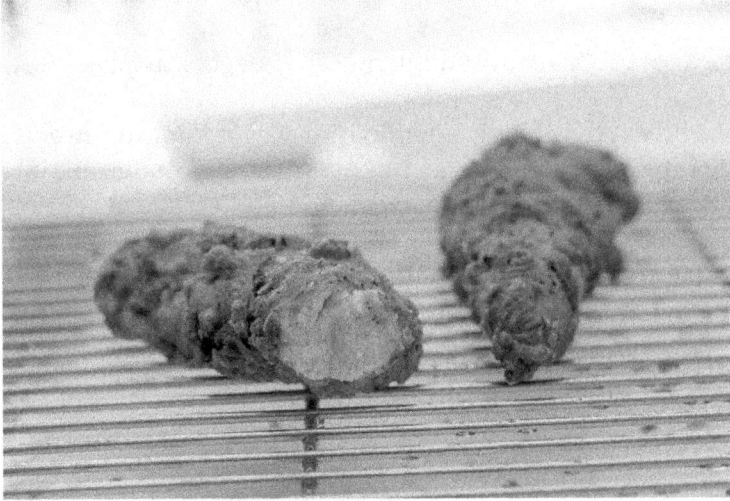

Serving: 6
Prep Time: 15 minutes
Cook Time: 30 minutes

Ingredients

- 2 pounds chicken breast, boneless and skinless
- 4 galric cloves, peeled and chopped
- 4 ounces clarified butter
- 1 cup fresh parmesan cheese, grated
- 2 tablespoons fresh thyme, chopped
- 1 teaspoon chili pepper flakes
- Salt and pepper to taste

How To

1. Pre-heat your oven to 350 degree F

2. Coat baking sheet with non-stick cooking spray

3. Take a saucepan and place it over medium heat

4. Add butter and let it melt, swirl the pan well to coat it

5. Stir in garlic and Saute for 15 minutes until fragrant, keep it on the side

6. Take another bowl and add thyme chili pepper, pepper, parmesan and stir

7. Rinse breast thoroughly and blot it dry with kitchen towel

8. Slice into 24 fingers and coat in the garlic and butter mix

9. Dredge the fingers in the cheese mix and arrange them on your baking sheet

10. Bake for 25-30 minutes until the fingers are golden brown

11. Transfer them to a cooling rack and allow them to cool

Nutrition (Per Serving)

- Calories: 370
- Fat: 20g
- Carbohydrates: 6g
- Protein: 40g

Clean Parsley And Chicken Breast

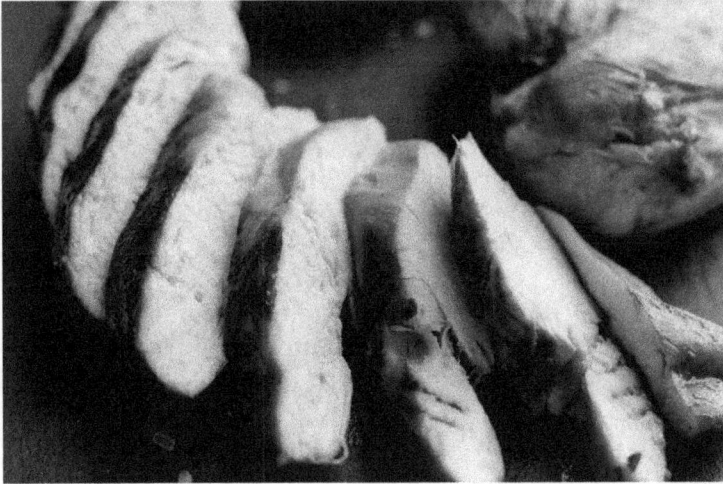

Serving: 4
Prep Time: 10 minutes
Cook Time: 40 minutes

Ingredients

- 1 tablespoon dry parsley
- 1 tablespoon dry basil
- 4 chicken breast halves, boneless and skinless
- ½ teaspoon salt
- ½ teaspoon red pepper flakes, crushed
- 2 tomatoes, sliced

How To

1. Pre-heat your oven to 350 degree F

2. Take a 9x13 inch baking dish and grease it up with cooking spray

3. Sprinkle 1 tablespoon of parsley, 1 teaspoon of basil and spread the mixture over your baking dish

4. Arrange the chicken breast halves over the dish and sprinkle garlic slices on top

5. Take a small bowl and add 1 teaspoon parsley, 1 teaspoon of basil, salt, basil, red pepper and mix well. Pour the mixture over the chicken breast

6. Top with tomato slices and cover, bake for 25 minutes

7. Remove the cover and bake for 15 minutes more

8. Serve and enjoy!

Nutrition (Per Serving)

- Calories: 150
- Fat: 4g
- Carbohydrates: 4g
- Protein: 25g

Chipotle Lettuce Chicken

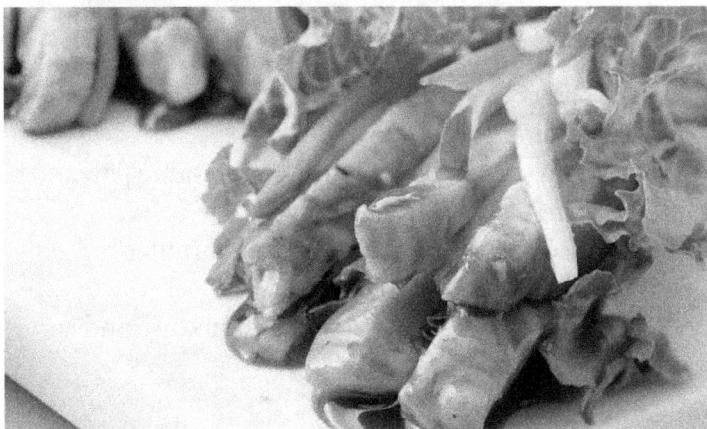

Serving: 6
Prep Time: 10 minutes
Cook Time: 25 minutes

Ingredients

- 1 pound chicken breast, cut into strips
- Splash of olive oil
- 1 red onion, finely sliced
- 14 ounces tomatoes
- 1 teaspoon chipotle, chopped
- ½ teaspoon cumin
- Pinch of sugar
- Lettuce as needed
- Fresh coriander leaves
- Jalapeno chilies, sliced
- Fresh tomato slices for garnish
- Lime wedges

How To

1. Take a non-stick frying pan and place it over medium heat

2. Add oil and heat it up

3. Add chicken and cook until brown

4. Keep the chicken on the side

5. Add tomatoes, sugar, chipotle, cumin to the same pan and simmer for 25 minutes until you have a nice sauce

6. Add chicken into the sauce and cook for 5 minutes

7. Transfer the mix to another place

8. Use lettuce wraps to take a portion of the mixture and serve with a squeeze of lemon

9. Enjoy!

Nutrition (Per Serving)

- Calories: 332
- Fat: 15g
- Carbohydrates: 13g
- Protein: 34g

Amazing Buffalo Lettuce Wraps

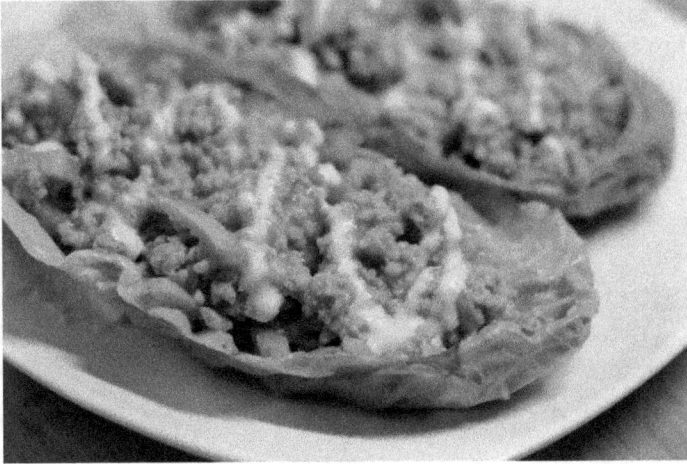

Serving: 2
Prep Time: 35 minutes
Cook Time: 10 minutes

Ingredients

- 3 chicken breast, boneless and cubed
- 20 slices of butter lettuce leaves
- ¾ cup cherry tomatoes, halved
- 1 avocado, chopped
- ¼ cup green onions, diced
- ½ a cup of ranch dressing
- ¾ cup hot sauce

How To

1. Take a mixing bowl and add chicken cubes and hot sauce, mix
2. Place in fridge and let it marinate for 30 minutes
3. Pre-heat your oven to 400 degree Fahrenheit
4. Place coated chicken on cookie pan and bake for 9 minutes
5. Assemble lettuce serving cups with equal amounts of lettuce, green onions, tomatoes, ranch dressing and cubed chicken
6. Serve and enjoy!

Nutrition(Per Serving)

- Calories: 106
- Fat: 6g
- Net Carbohydrates: 2g
- Protein: 5g

Balsamic Chicken

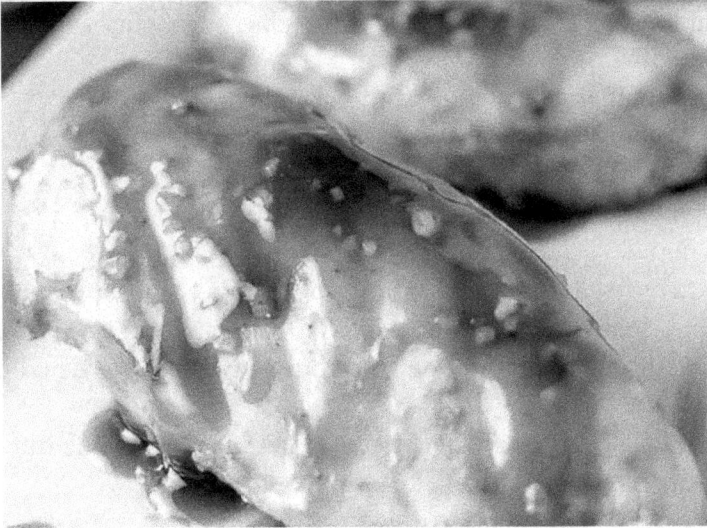

Serving: 6
Prep Time: 10 minutes
Cook Time: 25 minutes

Ingredients

- 6 chicken breast halves, skinless and boneless
- 1 teaspoon garlic salt
- Ground black pepper
- 2 tablespoons olive oil
- 1 onion, thinly sliced
- 14 and ½ ounces tomatoes, diced
- ½ cup balsamic vinegar
- 1 teaspoon dried basil
- 1 teaspoon dried oregano
- 1 teaspoon dried rosemary
- ½ teaspoon dried thyme

How To

1. Season both sides of your chicken breasts thoroughly with pepper and garlic salt

2. Take a skillet and place it over medium heat

3. Add some oil and cook your seasoned chicken for 3-4 minutes per side until the breasts are nicely browned

4. Add some onion and cook for another 3-4 minutes until the onions are browned

5. Pour the diced up tomatoes and balsamic vinegar over your chicken and season with some rosemary, basil, thyme and rosemary

6. Simmer the chicken for about 15 minutes until they are no longer pink

7. Take an instant read thermometer and check if the internal temperature gives a reading of 165 degree Fahrenheit

8. If yes, then you are good to go!

Nutrition (Per Serving)

- Calories: 196
- Fat: 7g
- Carbohydrates: 7g
- Protein: 23g

Fish and Seafood Recipes

Tilapia Broccoli Platter

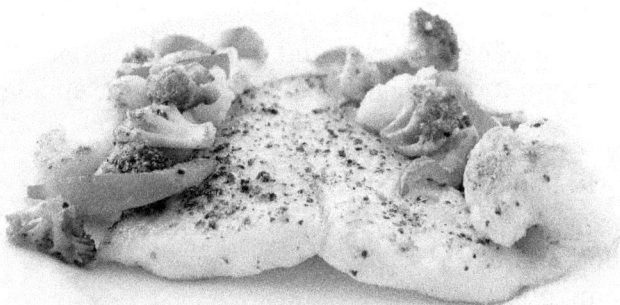

Serving: 2
Prep Time: 4 minutes
Cook Time: 14 minutes

Ingredients
- 6 ounce of tilapia, frozen
- 1 tablespoon of butter
- 1 tablespoon of garlic, minced
- 1 teaspoon of lemon pepper seasoning
- 1 cup of broccoli florets, fresh

How To

1. Pre-heat your oven to 350 degree F
2. Add fish in aluminum foil packets
3. Arrange broccoli around fish
4. Sprinkle lemon pepper on top
5. Close the packets and seal
6. Bake for 14 minutes
7. Take a bowl and add garlic and butter, mix well and keep the mixture on the side
8. Remove the packet from oven and transfer to platter
9. Place butter on top of the fish and broccoli, serve and enjoy!

Nutrition (Per Serving)

- Calories: 362
- Fat: 25g
- Carbohydrates: 2g
- Protein: 29g

Simple Baked Shrimp With Béchamel Sauce

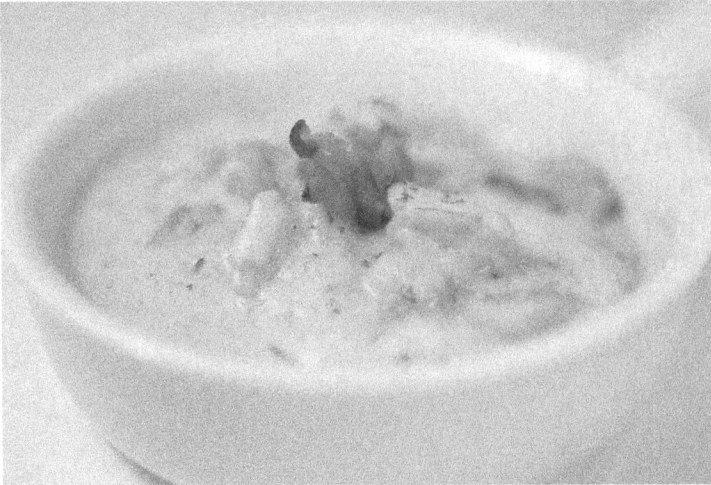

Serving: 4
Prep Time: 10 minutes
Cook Time: 5-7 minutes

Ingredients

- 6-7 ounces shrimp
- 1 ounce mozzarella
- 4 ounces béchamel sauce (recipe provided)
- 1 tablespoons ghee

How To

1. Cut boiled shrimp and transfer them to baking dish

2. Pour sauce on top

3. Bake for 5-7 minutes

4. Serve and enjoy!

Nutrition (Per Serving)

- Calories: 150
- Fat: 10g
- Carbohydrates: 2g
- Protein: 14g

Simple Sautéed Garlic And Parsley Scallops

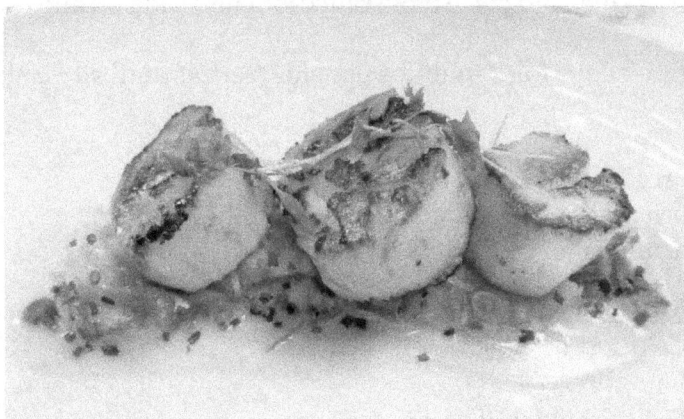

Serving: 4
Prep Time: 5 minutes
Cook Time: 25 minutes

<u>Ingredients</u>

- 8 tablespoons butter
- 2 garlic cloves, minced
- 16 large sea scallops
- Salt and pepper to taste
- 1 and ½ tablespoons olive oil

How To

1. Seasons scallops with salt and pepper
2. Take a skillet and place it over medium heat, add oil and let it heat up
3. Saute scallops for 2 minutes per side, repeat until all Scallops are cooked
4. Add butter to the skillet and let it melt
5. Stir in garlic and cook for 15 minutes
6. Return scallops to skillet and stir to coat
7. Serve and enjoy!

Nutrition (Per Serving)

- Calories: 417
- Fat: 31g
- Net Carbohydrates: 5g
- Protein: 29g

Mesmerizing Coconut Haddock

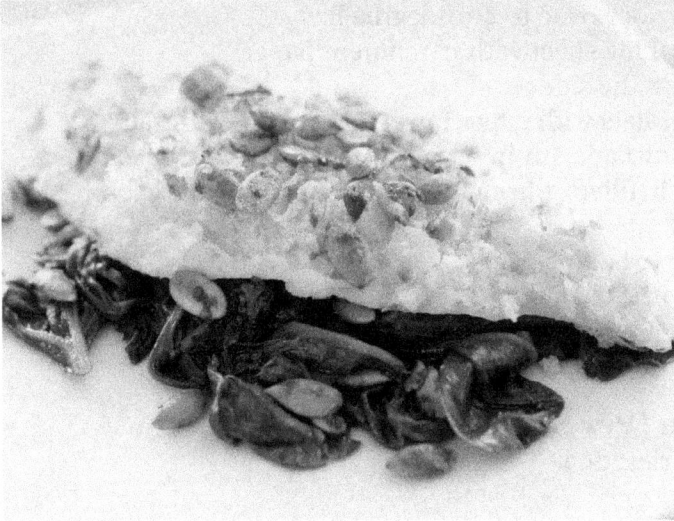

Serving: 3
Prep Time: 10 minutes
Cook Time: 12 minutes

Ingredients

- 4 haddock fillets, 5 ounces each, boneless
- 2 tablespoons coconut oil, melted
- 1 cup coconut, shredded and unsweetened
- ¼ cup hazelnuts, ground
- Salt to taste

How To

1. Pre-heat your oven to 400-degree F

2. Line a baking sheet with parchment paper

3. Keep it on the side

4. Pat fish fillets with paper towel and season with salt

5. Take a bowl and stir in hazelnuts and shredded coconut

6. Drag fish fillets through the coconut mix until both sides are coated well

7. Transfer to baking dish

8. Brush with coconut oil

9. Bake for about 12 minutes until flaky

10. Serve and enjoy!

Nutrition (Per Serving)

- Calories: 299
- Fat: 24g
- Carbohydrates: 1g
- Protein: 20g

"Salmon" Platter

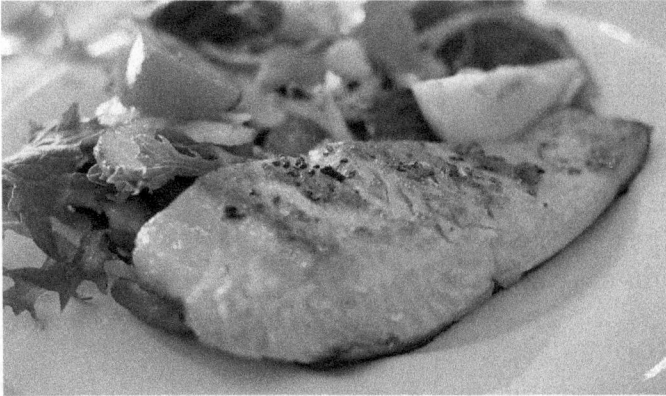

Serving: 3
Prep Time: 5 minute
Cook Time: 6 minutes

Ingredients

- ¾ cup of water
- Few sprigs of parsley, basil, tarragon, basil
- 1 pound of salmon , skin on
- 3 teaspoon of ghee
- ¼ teaspoon of salt
- ½ teaspoon of pepper
- ½ of a lemon, thinly sliced
- 1 whole carrot, julienned

How To

1. Set your pot to Saute mode and water and herbs
2. Place a steamer rack inside your pot and place salmon
3. Drizzle Ghee on top of the salmon and season with salt and pepper
4. Cover lemon slices
5. Lock up the lid and cook on HIGH pressure for 3 minutes
6. Release the pressure naturally over 10 minutes
7. Transfer the salmon to a serving platter
8. Set your pot to Saute mode and add vegetables
9. Cook for 1-2 minutes
10. Serve with vegetables and salmon
11. Enjoy!

Nutrition Values (Per Serving)

- Calories: 464
- Fat: 34g
- Carbohydrates: 3g
- Protein: 34g

Soups and Stews Recipes

Hearty Keto Chicken And Egg Soup

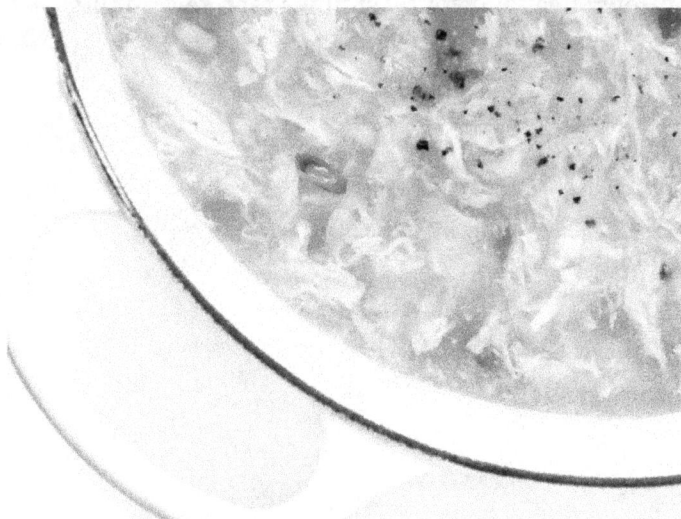

Serving: 2
Prep Time: 5 minutes
Cook Time: 10 minutes

Ingredients
- 1 and ½ cup chicken broth
- 2 whole eggs
- 1 teaspoon chili garlic paste
- 1 tablespoon bacon grease
- ½ a cube, chicken bouillon

How To

1. Take a stove top pan and place it over medium-high heat
2. Add chicken broth, bouillon cube, bacon grease and stir
3. Bring the mix to a boil
4. Mix in chili garlic paste
5. Take a bowl and whisk in eggs, add whisked egg to the pan
6. Lower down heat and gently simmer for a few minutes
7. Serve and enjoy!

Nutrition (Per Serving)

- Calories: 280
- Fat: 25g
- Carbohydrates: 3g
- Protein: 14g

Ingenious Eggplant Soup

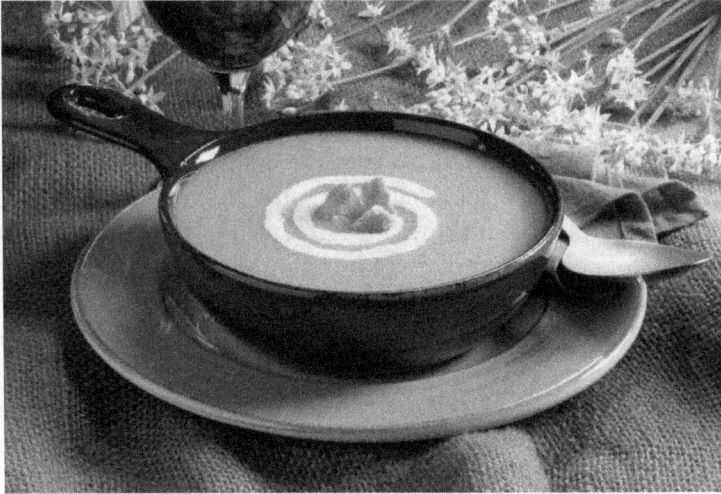

Serving: 8
Prep Time: 20 minutes
Cook Time: 15 minutes

Ingredients

- 1 large eggplant, washed and cubed
- 1 tomato, seeded and chopped
- 1 small onion, diced
- 2 tablespoons parsley, chopped
- 2 tablespoons extra virgin olive oil
- 2 tablespoons distilled white vinegar
- ½ cup parmesan cheese, crumbled
- Salt as needed

How To
1. Pre-heat your outdoor grill to medium-high
2. Pierce the eggplant a few times using a knife/fork
3. Cook the eggplants on your grill for about 15 minutes until they are charred
4. Keep it on the side and allow them to cool
5. Remove the skin from the eggplant and dice the pulp
6. Transfer the pulp to mixing bowl and add parsley, onion, tomato, olive oil, feta cheese and vinegar
7. Mix well and chill for 1 hour
8. Season with salt and enjoy!

Nutrition (Per Serving)
- Calories: 99
- Fat: 7g
- Carbohydrates: 7g
- Protein:3.4g

Amazing Roasted Carrot Soup

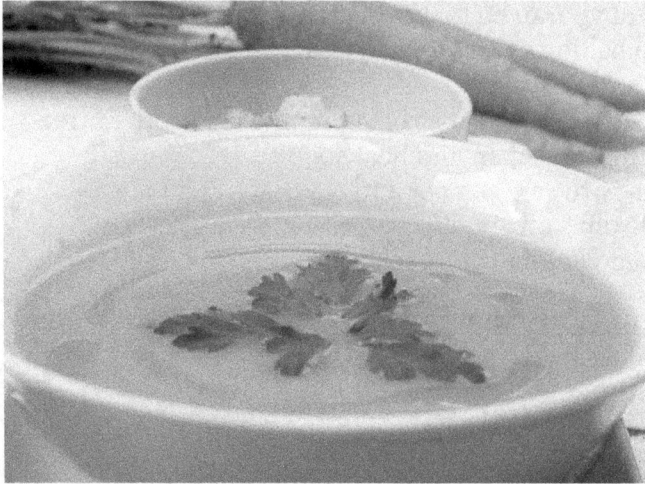

Serving: 4
Prep Time: 10 minutes
Cook Time: 50 minutes

Ingredients

- 8 large carrot,s washed and peeeld
- 6 tablespoons olive oil
- 1 quart broth
- Cayenne pepper to taste
- Salt and pepper to taste

How To

1. Pre-heat your oven to 425 degree F

2. Take a baking sheet and add carrots, drizzle olive oil and roast for 30-45 minutes

3. Put roasted carrots into blender and add broth, puree

4. Pour into saucepan and heat soup

5. Season with salt, pepper and cayenne

6. Drizzle olive oil

7. Serve and enjoy!

Nutrition (Per Serving)

- Calories: 222
- Fat: 18g
- Net Carbohydrates: 7g
- Protein: 5g

The Brussels's Fever

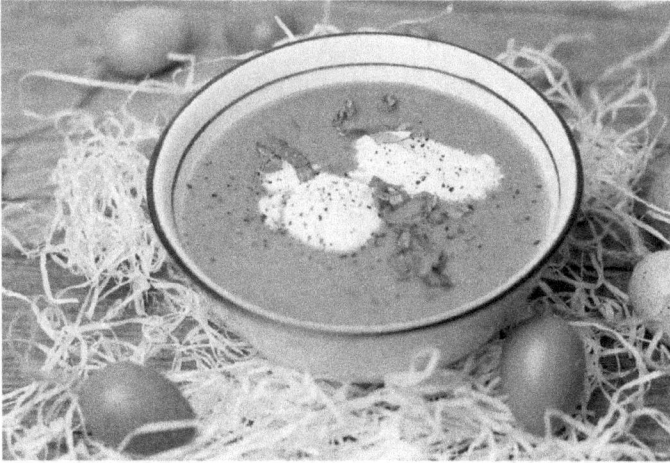

Serving: 4
Prep Time: 10 minutes
Cook Time: 20 minutes

Ingredients

- 2 tablespoons olive oil
- 1 yellow onion, chopped
- 2 pounds Brussels sprouts, trimmed and halved
- 4 cups chicken stock
- ¼ cup coconut cream

How To

1. Take a pot and place it over medium heat

2. Add oil and let it heat up

3. Add onion and stir cook for 3 minutes

4. Add Brussels sprouts and stir, cook for 2 minutes

5. Add stock and black pepper, stir and bring to a simmer

6. Cook for 20 minutes more

7. Use an immersion blender to make the soup creamy

8. Add coconut cream and stir well

9. Ladle into soup bowls and serve

10. Enjoy!

Nutrition (Per Serving)

- Calories: 200
- Fat: 11g
- Carbohydrates: 6g
- Protein: 11g

Curious Roasted Garlic Soup

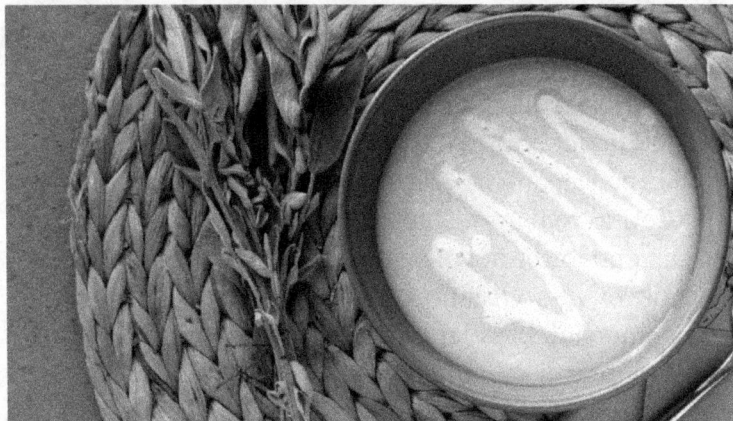

Serving: 10
Prep Time: 10 minutes
Cook Time: 60 minutes

Ingredients

- 1 tablespoons olive oil
- 2 bulbs garlic, peeled
- 3 shallots, chopped
- 1 large head cauliflower, chopped
- 6 cups vegetable broth
- Salt and pepper to taste

How To

1. Pre-heat your oven to 400 degree F
2. Slice ¼ inch top of garlic bulb and place it in an aluminum foil
3. Grease with olive oil and roast in oven for 35 minutes
4. Squeeze flesh out of the roasted garlic
5. Heat oil in saucepan and add shallots, Saute for 6 minutes
6. Add garlic and remaining ingredients
7. Cover pan and lower down heat to low
8. Let it cook for 15-20 minutes
9. Use an immersion blender to puree the mixture
10. Season soup with salt and pepper
11. Serve and enjoy!

Nutrition (Per Serving)

- Calories: 142
- Fat: 8g
- Carbohydrates: 3.4g
- Protein: 4g

Desserts Recipes

Almond Butter Cup Cookies

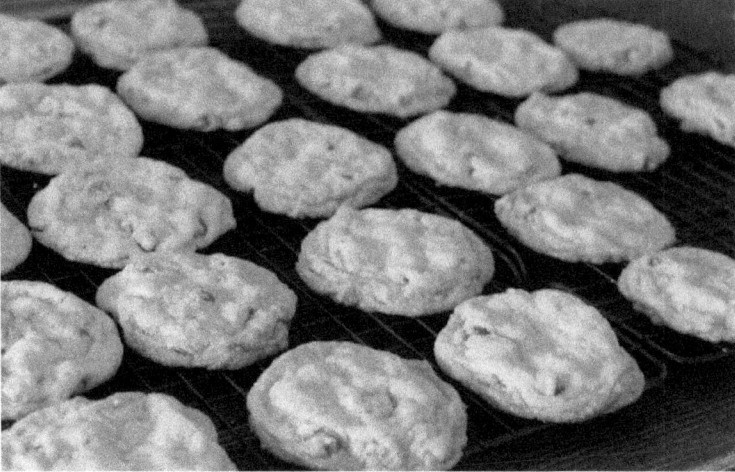

Serving: 4
Prep Time: 10 minutes
Cook Time: 90 minutes

Ingredients

- 1 cup almond butter
- ½ cup coconut crystals
- 1 teaspoon vanilla bean extract
- ¼ teaspoon almond extract
- 2 whole eggs
- ½ cup almond flour, blanched
- 2 tablespoons coconut flour
- ¼ teaspoon salt
- 1 cup dark chocolate, chopped, unsweetened

How To
1. Pre-heat your oven to 350 degree F
2. Prepare baking sheet by lightly greasing it with coconut oil
3. Add crystal, almond butter, eggs, almond extract and vanilla extract in a medium bowl
4. Mix well
5. Take another bowl and add flours, salt and mix
6. Add the flour mix to the bowl with wet ingredients and stir until combined
7. Form golf ball sized cookies and form them into peanut butter cups
8. Place cookies on baking sheet and let them bake for 12 minutes
9. Chill for 30 minutes in refrigerators
10. Melt chocolate over medium heat in double boiler and cool for 15 minutes, pour chocolate over chilled cookies
11. Serve and enjoy!

Nutrition (Per Serving)
- Calories: 173
- Fat: 11g
- Carbohydrates: 5g
- Protein: 4g

Lovely Pumpkin Buns

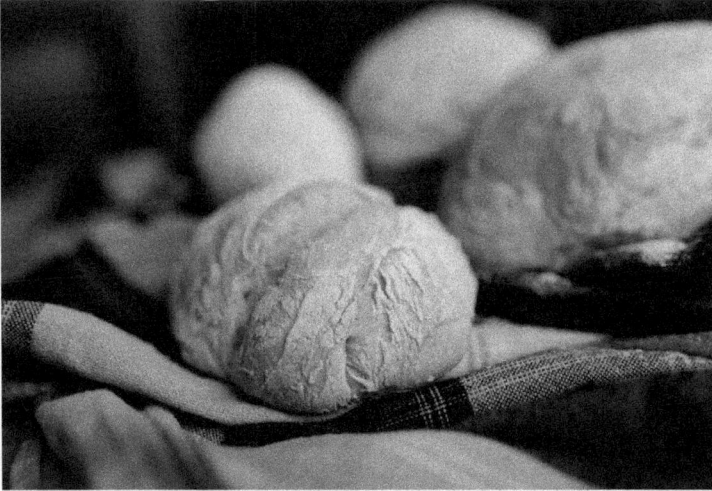

Serving: 10
Prep Time: 10 minutes
Cook Time: 50 minutes

Ingredients

- ½ cup coconut flour
- 1 and ½ cups almond flour
- ½ cup ground flax seeds
- 1 teaspoon onion powder
- 1 teaspoon garlic powder
- 1 teaspoon baking soda
- 2 teaspoon cream of tartar
- 5 tablespoons sesame seeds
- 1 teaspoons salt

Wet Ingredients

- 2 Eggs
- 6 egg whites
- 1 cup warm water
- 1/3 cup Psyllium husk powder

How To
1. Pre-heat your oven to 350 degree F
2. Take a baking tray and line it up with parchment paper, keep it on the side
3. Take a bowl and mix in dry ingredients, mix it well
4. Take another bowl and whisk in eggs, water and husk
5. Mix well until smooth
6. Slowly add dry ingredients into wet ingredients bowl
7. Keep mixing until you have an even dough
8. Knead dough until smooth and roll dough into buns, arrange them on your baking tray
9. Bake for 50 minutes
10. Once done, remove from oven and let them cool. Serve!

Nutrition (Per Serving)
- Calories: 189
- Fat: 13g
- Carbohydrates: 6g
- Protein: 10g

Gingerbread Keto Muffins

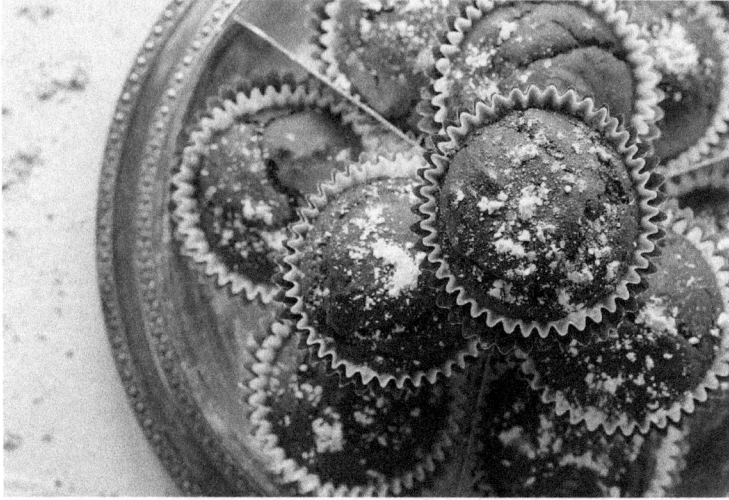

Serving: 6
Prep Time: 10 minutes
Cook Time: 10-15 minutes

Ingredients

- 1 tablespoon ground flaxseed
- 6 tablespoons coconut milk
- 1 tablespoon apple cider vinegar
- ½ cup peanut butter
- 2 tablespoons gingerbread spice blend
- 1 teaspoon baking powder
- 1 teaspoon vanilla extract
- 2 tablespoons Swerve

How To
1. Pre-heat your oven to 350 degree F
2. Take a bowl and add flaxseed, salt, vanilla, sweetener, spices and non-dairy milk
3. Keep it on the side
4. Add peanut butter, baking powder and keep mixing
5. Stir well
6. Spoon batter into muffin liners and bake for 30 minutes
7. Let them cool and serve
8. Enjoy!

Nutrition (Per Serving)
- Calories: 283
- Fat: 23g
- Carbohydrates: 13g
- Protein: 11g

Sensational Lemonade Fat Bomb

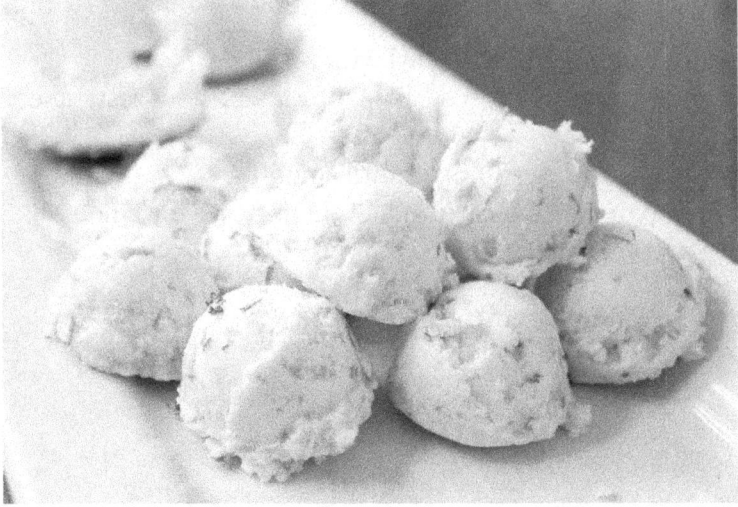

Serving: 2
Prep Time: 2 hours
Cook Time: Nil

Ingredients

- ½ a lemon
- 4 ounces cream cheese
- 2 ounces butter
- Salt to taste
- 2 teaspoon natural sweetener

How To

1. Take a fin grater and zest lemon

2. Squeeze lemon juice into bowl with zest

3. Add butter, cream cheese in a bowl and add zest, juice, salt, sweetener

4. Mix well using a hand mixer until smooth

5. Spoon mixture into molds and let them freeze for 2 hours

6. Serve and enjoy!

Nutrition (Per Serving)

- Calories: 404
- Fat: 43g
- Carbohydrates: 4g
- Protein: 4g

The Easy "No Bake" Fudge

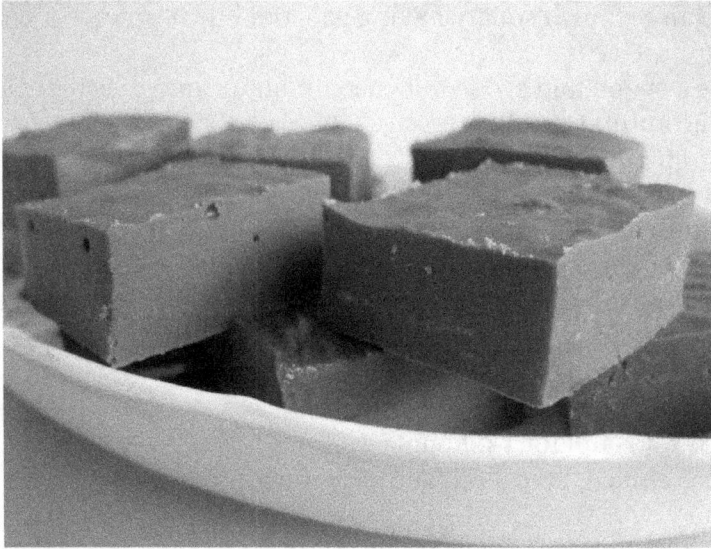

Serving: 25
Prep Time: 15 minutes + chill time
Cook Time: 5 minutes

Ingredients

- 1 and ¾ cups coconut butter
- 1 cup pumpkin puree
- 1 teaspoon ground cinnamon
- ¼ teaspoon ground nutmeg
- 1 tablespoon coconut oil

How To

1. Take an 8x8 inch square baking pan and line it up with aluminum foil

2. Take a spoon and scoop out coconut butter into a heated pan and allow the butter to melt

3. Keep stirring well and remove the heat once fully melted

4. Add spices and pumpkin and keep straining until you have a grain like texture

5. Add coconut oil and keep stirring to incorporate everything

6. Scoop the mixture into your baking pan and evenly distribute it

7. Place a wax paper on top of the mixture and press gently to straighten the top

8. Remove the paper and discard

9. Allow it to chill for 1-2 hours

10. Once chilled, take it out and slice it up into pieces

11. Enjoy!

Nutrition (Per Serving)

- Calories: 120
- Fat: 10g
- Carbohydrates: 5g
- Protein: 1.2g

Vegan and Vegetarian Recipes

Chipotle Kale Chips

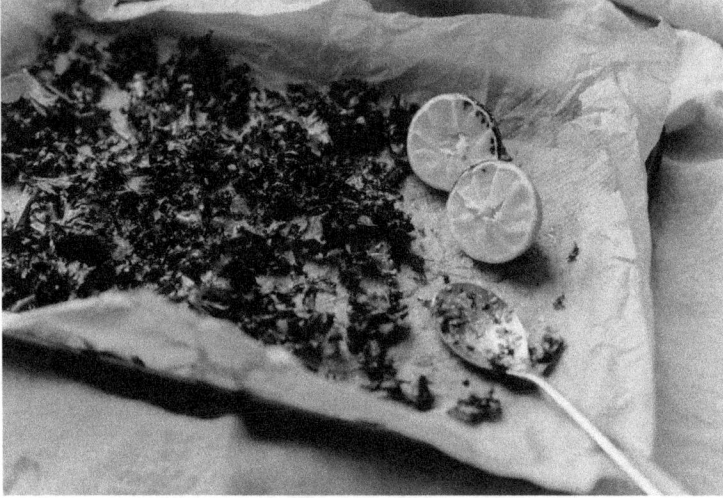

Serving: 4
Prep Time: 4 minutes
Cook Time: 29 minutes

Ingredients

- 2 large bunch kale, chopped into 4 pieces and stemmed
- 1 tablespoon olive oil
- 1/8 teaspoon salt
- 1 teaspoon chipotle powder
- ¼ cup parmesan cheese, shredded

How To

1. Wash kale thoroughly and dry, cut into 4 inch pieces
2. Pre-heat your oven to 250 degree F
3. Take a baking sheet and line with parchment paper
4. Take a bowl and add kale, coat the kale with olive oil, chipotle and cheese
5. Transfer the mix to baking sheet
6. Bake for 19 minutes and check the crispiness
7. If you need more crispiness, bake for 9 minutes more
8. Serve and enjoy!

Nutrition (Per Serving)

- Calories: 37
- Fat: 3g
- Carbohydrates: 2g
- Protein: 1g

Classic Guacamole

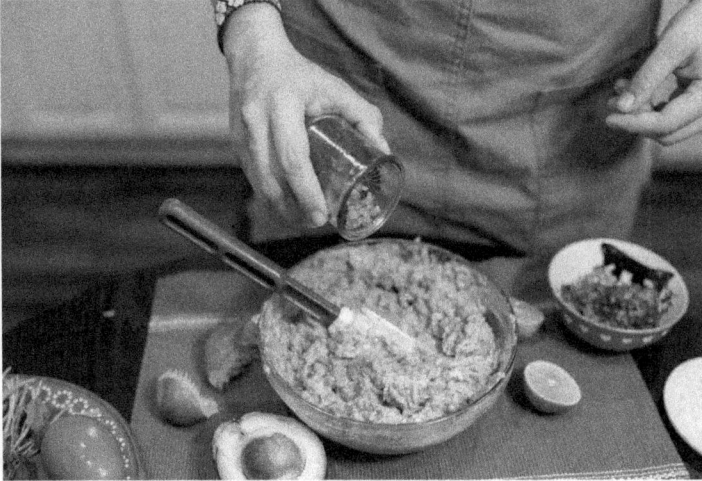

Serving: 6
Prep Time: 15 minutes
Cook Time: Nil

Ingredients

- 3 large ripe avocados
- 1 large red onion, peeled and diced
- 4 tablespoon of freshly squeeze lime juice
- Salt as needed
- Freshly ground black pepper as needed
- Cayenne pepper as needed

How To

1. Halve the avocados and discard stone

2. Scoop flesh from 3 avocado halves and transfer to a large bowl

3. Mash using fork

4. Add 2 tablespoon of lime juice and mix

5. Dice the remaining avocado flesh (remaining half) and transfer to another bowl

6. Add remaining juice and toss

7. Add diced flesh with the mashed flesh and mix

8. Add chopped onions and toss

9. Season with salt, pepper and cayenne pepper

10. Serve and enjoy!

Nutrition (Per Serving)

- Calories: 172
- Fat: 15g
- Carbohydrates: 11g
- Protein: 2g

Astonishingly Simple Lettuce Salad

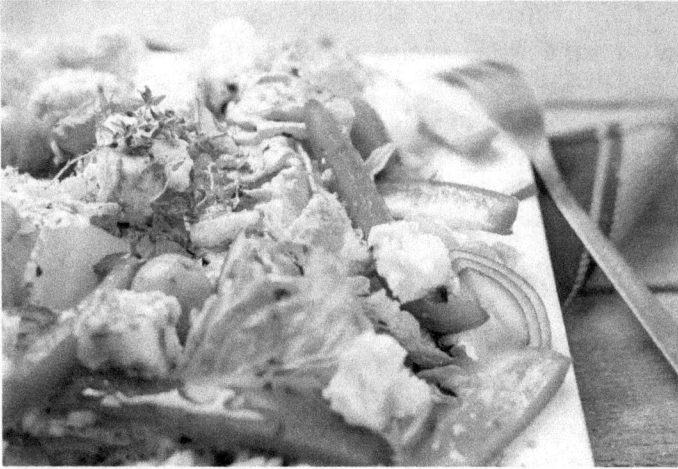

Serving: 2
Prep Time: 10 minutes
Cook Time: Nil minutes

Ingredients
- 2 ounces Romaine lettuce
- ½ ounce butter
- 1 ounce Adam cheese, sliced
- ½ avocado, sliced
- 1 cherry tomato, sliced
- 1 red bell pepper, sliced

How To

1. Add butter on top of each lettuce leaves

2. Add alternating layers of cheese, avocado, tomato slices

3. Serve and enjoy!

Nutrition (Per Serving)

- Calories: 104
- Fat: 14g
- Carbohydrates: 4g
- Protein: 4g

Light Egg Salad

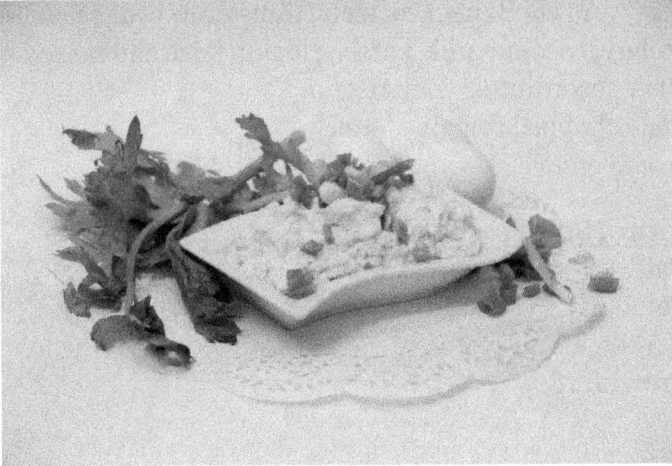

Serving: 4
Prep Time: 5 minutes
Cook Time: 15 minutes

Ingredients

- 3 hard-boiled eggs, cooled
- 2 tablepoons celery, diced
- 3 tablespoon canned coconut milk
- 1 tablesooon parsley, chopped
- 1 teaspoon fresh lemon juice
- Salt and pepper as needed
- 1 and ½ cups romain lettuce, chopped

How To

1. Peel eggs and chop them coarsely, transfer to your salad bowl

2. Add celery, coconut milk, parsley, lemon juice and season with salt and pepper according to your taste

3. Sprinkle chopped romaine lettuce

4. Serve and enjoy!

Nutrition (Per Serving)

- Calories: 300
- Fat: 24g
- Carbohydrates: 3g
- Protein: 18g

Buttery Green Cabbage

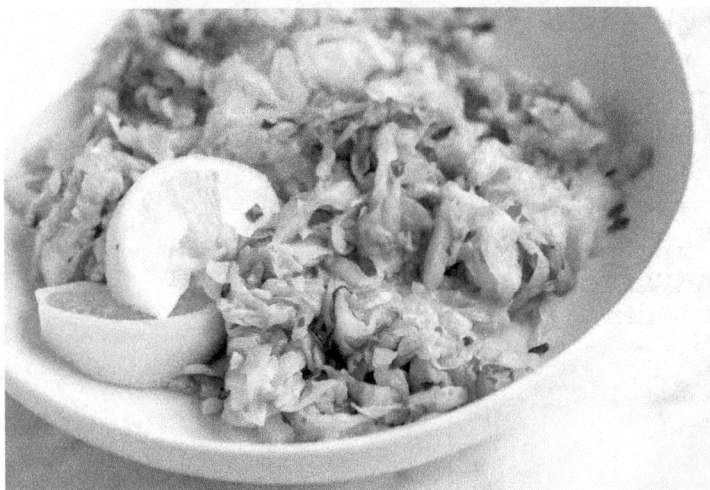

Serving: 4
Prep Time: 10 minutes
Cook Time: 15 minutes

Ingredients

- 1 and ½ pounds shredded green cabbage
- 3 ounces butter
- Salt and pepper to taste
- 1 dollop, whipped cream

How To

1. Take a large skillet and place it over medium heat

2. Add butter and melt

3. Stir in cabbage and Saute for 15 minutes

4. Season accordingly

5. Serve with a dollop of cream

6. Enjoy!

Nutrition (Per Serving)

- Calories: 199
- Fat: 17g
- Carbohydrates: 10g
- Protein: 3g

Refreshing Drinks And Smoothies

The Refreshing Nut Smoothie

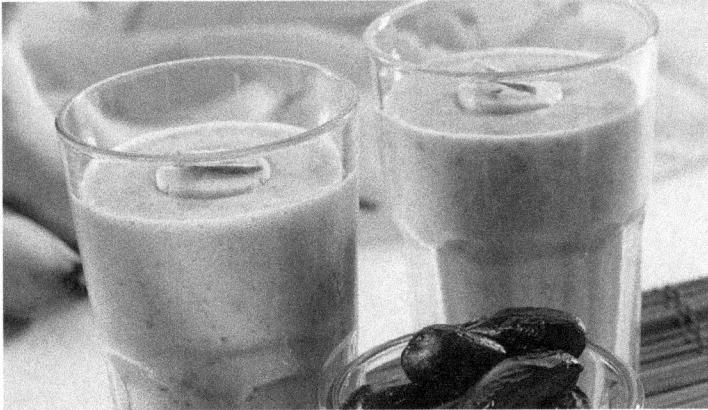

Serving: 1
Prep Time: 10 minutes

Ingredients:
- 1 tablespoon chia seeds
- 2 cups water
- 1 ounces Macadamia Nuts
- 1-2 packets Stevia, optional
- 1 ounces Hazelnut

Directions:
1. Add all the listed ingredients to a blender.
2. Blend on high until smooth and creamy.
3. Enjoy your smoothie.

Nutritional Contents:

- Calories: 452
- Fat: 43g
- Carbohydrates: 15g
- Protein: 9g

Salted Macadamia Choco Smoothie

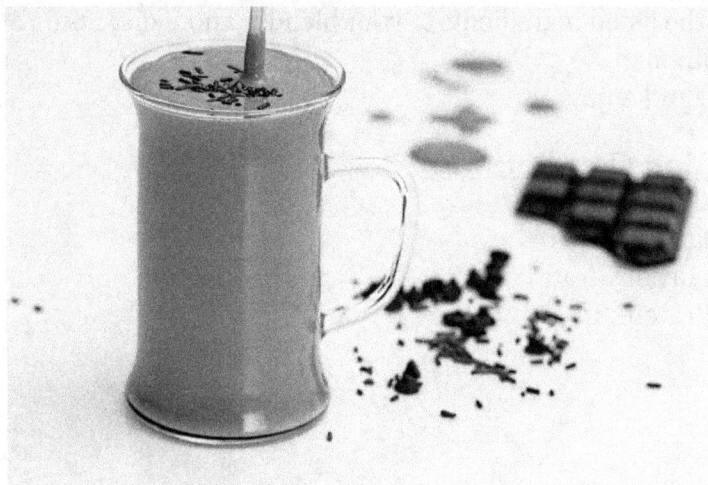

Serving: 1
Prep Time: 5 minutes
Cook Time: Nil

<u>Ingredients</u>

- 2 tablespoons macadamia nuts, salted
- 1/3 cup chocolate whey protein powder, low carb
- 1 cup almond milk, unsweetened

How To

1. Add the listed ingredients to your blender and blend until you have a smooth mixture

2. Chill and enjoy!

Nutrition (Per Serving)

- Calories: 165
- Fat: 2g
- Carbohydrates: 1g
- Protein: 12g

Chia And Coffee Blend

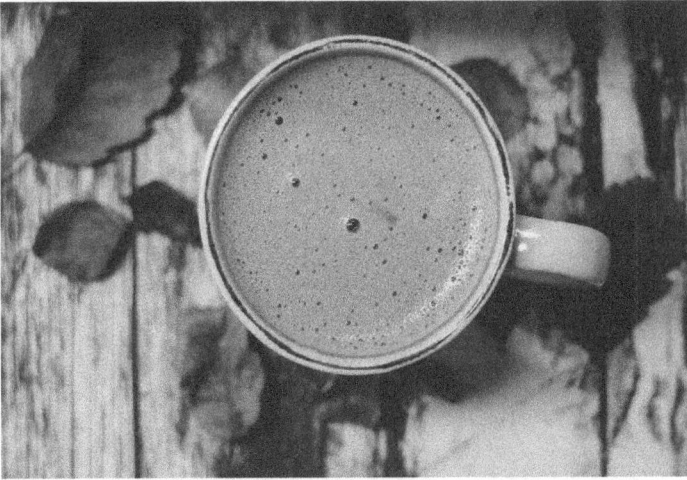

Serving: 1
Prep Time: 10 minutes

Ingredients:

- 1 tablespoon chia seeds
- 2 cups stongly brewed coffee, chilled
- 1 ounce Macadamia Nuts
- 1-2 packets Stevia, optional
- 1 tablespoon MCT oil

Directions:

1. Add all the listed ingredients to a blender.
2. Blend on high until smooth and creamy.
3. Enjoy your smoothie.

Nutritional Contents:

- Calories: 395
- Fat: 39g
- Carbohydrates: 11g
- Protein: 5.2g

Cilantro And Citrus Glass

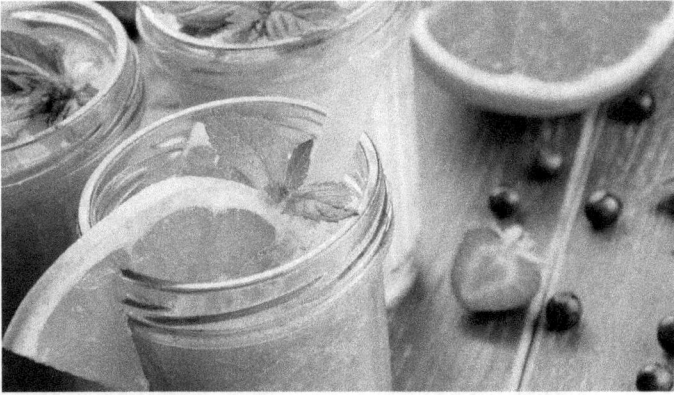

Serving: 2
Prep Time: 5 minutes

- ½ cup ice
- 2 cups arugula
- ½ cup celery, diced
- 1 grapefruit, peeled and segmented
- 1 handful fresh cilantro leaves, chopped
- ½ lemon, juiced
- ½ cup of water

Directions

1. Add all the ingredients except vegetables/fruits first
2. Blend until smooth
3. Add the vegetable/fruits
4. Blend until smooth
5. Add a few ice cubes and serve the smoothie
6. Enjoy!
7.

Nutrition Values

- Calories: 75
- Fat: 1g
- Carbohydrates: 16g
- Protein: 3g

The Wild Matcha Delight

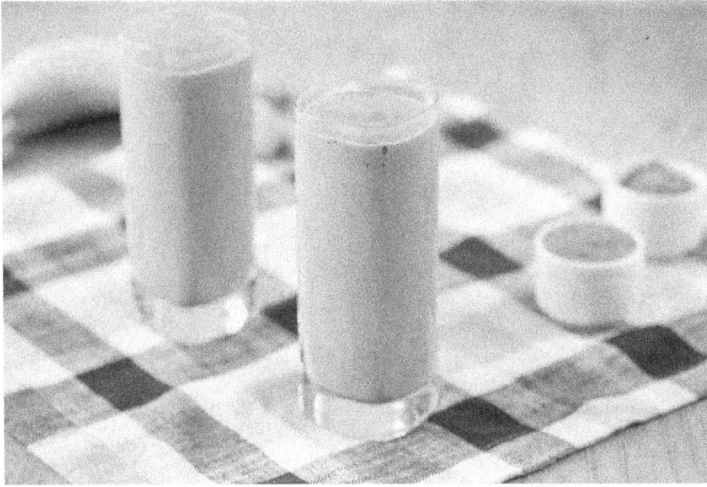

Serving: 2
Prep Time: 5 minutes
Ingredients

- 1 cup unsweetened coconut milk
- 1 teaspoon matcha powder
- ½ teaspoon cinnamon
- 1 cup baby spinach, chopped
- 1 cup wild blueberries, frozen

Directions

1. Add all the ingredients except vegetables/fruits first
2. Blend until smooth
3. Add the vegetable/fruits
4. Blend until smooth
5. Add a few ice cubes and serve the smoothie
6. Enjoy!

Nutrition Values

- Calories: 130
- Fat: 3g
- Carbohydrates: 17g
- Protein: 5g

CPSIA information can be obtained
at www.ICGtesting.com
Printed in the USA
BVHW042324310521
608489BV00016B/2752

9 781802 838367